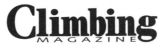

Home Climbing Gyms

How to build and use

By Randy Leavitt
Illustrated by John McMullen
Photos by Anthony Scoggins

PRIMEDIA/Cowles Enthusiast Media/Climbing Magazine
1101 Village Road, LL-1-B
Carbondale, Colorado 81623
970-963-9449
First Printing 1998

Library of Congress Catalog Card Number

By Randy Leavitt
Illustrated by John McMullen
Photos by Anthony Scoggins
ISBN 1-887216-11-1

Printed in the United States of America
10   9   8   7   6   5   4   3   2   1

Table of contents

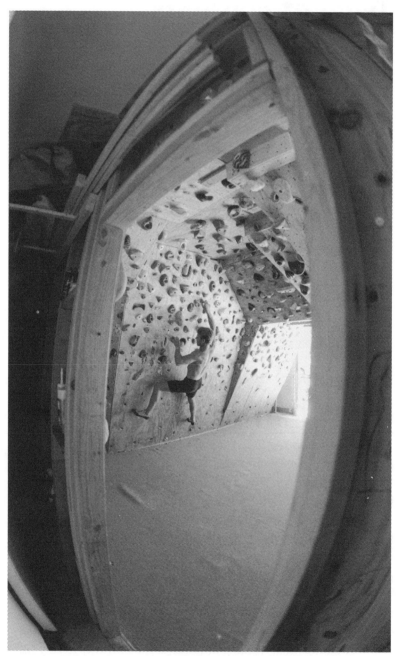

Want to improve your rock-climbing performance? Build and use a home gym.

Why and where to build a home gym

A home climbing gym is your most valuable asset for enjoying and excelling in rock climbing. We should feel fortunate because few other adventure sports let you practice at home. Take surfing — ever try to build a wave machine in your garage? What about skydiving? You might balk at the prospect of building a vertical wind tunnel where your truck should be parked. Build a rock-climbing gym in your own home, because doing so is inexpensive, easy, and because you can.

Rock climbing at your maximum standard requires a non-stop approach to fitness. A month of non-climbing is enough to drastically affect your performance. Unless you live next to a great year-round climbing area, training at home is the only way to stay fit.

A home climbing gym will improve your strength, endurance, and technique. You can set specific problems to attack your weaknesses and establish routes that remain as permanent benchmarks for your progress. Because you can rearrange the holds in your gym, you can always find new challenges and stay motivated to train.

A home gym will help you to utilize your time better. Many of the hours you used to spend driving to local bouldering areas, commercial walls, and distant crags will now be spent in your gym. You can even mow your lawn between climbs.

Creating a positive social environment is another reason to build a gym. I have fond memories of hanging out in the air-conditioned comfort of my San Diego climbing gym, spending quality time with friends while the summer sun baked the life out of everything outside.

Most of all, your gym will make the time you do spend on real rock much more productive and enjoyable. You will feel fitter, more relaxed, and ready for your next project. So get ready and let your imagination fly. You will never look at your garage, basement, attic, or spare room the same way again.

Location, location

The ideal location for your home gym is a four-car garage with a 10-foot ceiling. If you don't have this posh facility, don't despair — you can put an effective home gym in some very surprising places. Tony Yaniro once built one in the bedroom of his second-floor apartment in Las Vegas. Tony's subsequent successes on 5.14s at the limestone of nearby Mount Charleston demonstrated that even three sheets of plywood can change life for the better.

A bedroom "woody" is great, but a garage, by virtue of being open and typically of unfinished interior construction, is the best choice, so let's start there. The garage is usually separated from the house, so the noise of your feet hitting the walls and floor or your CD player blasting won't distract your family. Chalk dust isn't much of a problem, especially if you don't mind some white powder on your shiny black car. (If your gym is well designed, you can still park your car(s) and your storage space will increase.) Finally, your oddball pastime is hidden from the neighbors and doesn't compromise your living space.

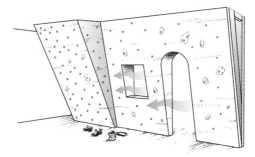

1-1. Design your wall so that it takes advantage of existing ventilation and lighting, such as windows and doors.

Besides a garage, there are other options:

Basement: Often good. Out of the way; temperate in summer and winter. Common problems include lack of height, natural lighting, and ventilation.

Attic: OK. Noise carries downstairs, and they're often hot and stuffy.

Interior room of house: Not ideal, but better than nothing. Chalk dust is always a problem; you can minimize this by using chalk balls and/or an air cleaner.

Exterior wall: Poor. You can't control the environment, attain proper lighting, or keep the elements from deteriorating the structure, panels, and holds. For these reasons, exterior walls are not recommended nor are they discussed in this book.

Regardless of where you decide to build your wall, consider a ceiling height of eight feet and a width of eight feet the minimums. Depth — the distance from the base of your wall to the farthest point onto which you might fall — should be at least 10 feet. Go less than that and you'll risk slamming into the wall or obstructions behind you when you go pinwheeling off of your problem.

A hot, dingy gym leads to uninspired climbing. Given a choice, choose a room with windows and cross ventilation. If you build your wall in front of existing doors and windows, consider "cut outs" to maximize the natural light and ventilation (figure 1-1). Don't overlook the predominant breezes in your area and the path of the sun. It is best to plan for the hottest days, rather than the coldest (i.e. don't face a cut-out to the east if you plan to climb mostly in the mornings). Artificial lights can be rigged anywhere, while fans and air conditioning can replace or supplement natural ventilation.

Construction basics

Climbing walls require only the most rudimentary construction skills. If you can swing a hammer, work a drill and circular saw, and operate a tape measure you have all of the skills you'll need.

Most climbers are familiar with the materials you'll use for your wall, but if you are new to the sport, know now that you'll be using plain-Jane plywood for the wall surface, and that the holds are made of plastic, though several companies offer real-rock counterparts. Either way, the holds bolt to the wall via threaded "T" nuts; moving them around is as simple as turning a wrench.

How much damage will your wall do to the room you build it in? In most cases you'll screw or nail the climbing-wall framing to the room's existing two-by-four wall studs, which are often covered over with drywall, which you'll either have to tear out or nail and screw through. Damage either way. Preferably, your room will be unfinished and the wall studs exposed. You can also anchor a gym to masonry, using your trusty hammer drill and masonry bolts, so don't rule out cinderblock, concrete-slab, or brick-walled rooms, though patching will be difficult should you ever remove the wall. If you don't have suitable anchor points, or are worried about getting back your renter's deposit, you can build a free-standing wall, but more on that later.

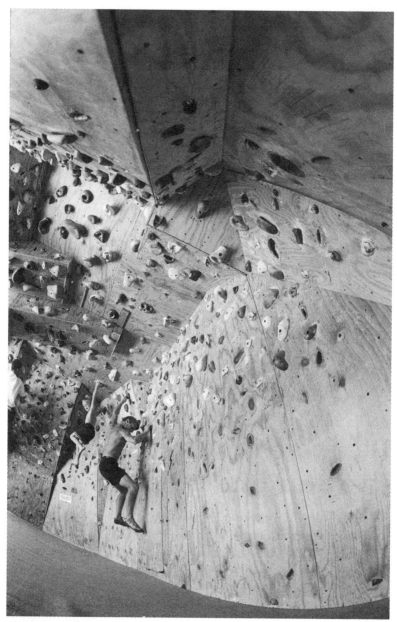

A well-thought-out wall provides a variety of angles and features that will keep you motivated for years to come.

Planning your climbing features and gym

The main features you choose for your gym will influence the overall design. Consider the following features as food for thought:

Standard-issue steep bouldering wall. This feature (figure 2-2, next page) is the basis for most home gyms due to ease of construction. The ideal angle is between 30 and 45 degrees overhanging — steep enough to throw weight onto your arms, but not so steep that you can't effectively train footwork. Vertical walls

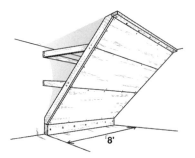

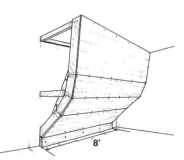

2-2. If your framing skills are minimal, start out with the easy-to-build, standard-issue 45-degree-overhanging bouldering wall.

2-3. Convex walls develop your abs and footwork by continually forcing you to pull in with your feet.

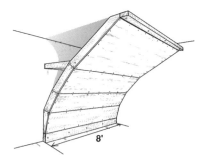

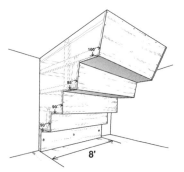

2-4. Concave walls let you suck in your hips and "sit" over your feet, making them less effective training devices than convex walls.

2-5. A stair-step wall will simulate the sort of blocky, overhanging climbing you'll find at Utah's American Fork or Colorado's Rifle canyons.

are virtually worthless. The standard-issue, steep bouldering wall is best built at least eight feet wide. With a nine-foot ceiling, the angle of the board will give you approximately 12 feet of upward climbing. If you have the space for two standard-issue bouldering walls, build one at 45 degrees and the other at 30 degrees.

Convex wall. This feature (figure 2-3) bows out and simulates the sort of climbing you find at Buoux, France. Your feet are on a steeper ground than your hands, so the wall promotes good, careful footwork and also gets you pumped. Convex walls require a ceiling of at least nine feet.

Concave wall. This is the inverse of the convex wall — it bows in (figure 2-4). It is less effective for training as you can often suck your hips into the wall and rest. Nevertheless, a concave wall

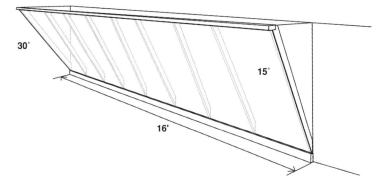

2-6. A bending wall requires complicated framing, but offers a continuous angle change that is akin to real rock – worth it if you're an adept carpenter.

provides interesting movement and, because it offers more climbing surface than a flat wall, will work in a gym with a relatively low seven-foot ceiling.

Stair-step wall. An upside-down staircase design (figure 2-5) simulates blocky, overhanging climbing, like that at American Fork, Utah. A bonus is that the back of a stair-step wall provides great shelf-like storage space.

Bending wall. If you have a long, traversing section (minimum 16 feet), you can start with one angle at one end (say 15 degrees), and build the wall progressively steeper (say to 30 degrees) toward the other end (figure 2-6). A bending

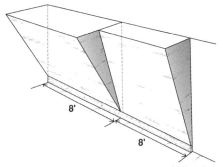

2-7. The multiple-angle wall serves the same function as a bending wall, but is easier to design and build.

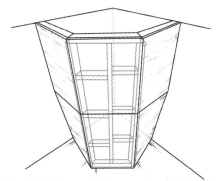

2-8. A ship's-bow wall takes an otherwise mundane corner, and adds an element of interest and difficulty.

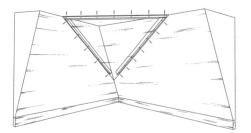

2-9. Triangular corner inserts yield interesting angle changes, and prevent you from "cheating" stem rests.

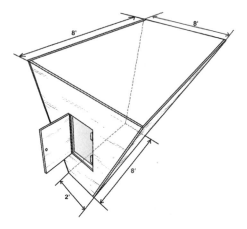

2-10. Island structures make ideal storage units.

wall is more difficult to build than a flat-paneled wall, but is fun and realistic because, like most rock, it has continuous rather than abrupt angle changes.

Multi-angle wall. You can use transition aretes to create several angles as you traverse across a wall (figure 2-7). This is much easier to build than a bending wall, and better suited for narrower areas (less than 16 feet wide).

Ship's-bow wall. This resembles the squared-off bow of a ship, and is a great feature to fill an inside corner (figure 2-8). It will add interest, cool moves, and mitigate stem rests (a common problem with inside corners).

Triangle insert. These flat, triangular, overhanging climbing panels can also be placed over inside corners, and are another good way to mitigate dreaded stem rests (figure 2-9).

Island. In a gym with 800 square feet of floor space or more, consider building a freestanding column at its center (figure 2-10). The island will resemble a wedge of cheese, having a small base with overhanging sides. An island gives you an area to climb to and around, rather than just aimlessly climbing across a large roof. It also increases your storage space.

Genie. If your automatic garage door opener or other essential device is built into a ceiling, you can enclose it with a Genie, a box-like feature that doesn't hinder the device's function (figure 2-11). This weird, hanging-down roof feature is fun to negotiate, so you might also consider building a Genie into any large section of roof.

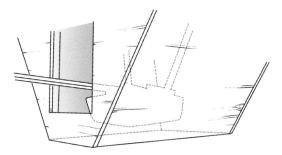

2-11. Cover your garage-door opener with a "Genie" and you'll protect it, plus create an interesting and climbable feature.

Campus board. This is a power-training device, consisting of a 12- to 15-degree-overhanging wall with evenly spaced wooden rungs (figure 2-12). The wall should be at least four feet high (preferably five or six) and undercut at the bottom so you can hang from the lowest rung with your legs slightly bent. From this hanging position, you make a series of footless dynos to ascend the wall. (See "Big man on campus," *Climbing* No. 158, for tips on building and training on a campus board.)

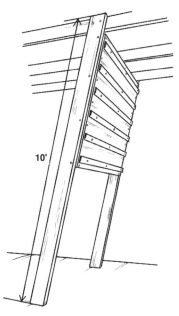

2-12. The campus board is the most effective way to develop your explosive power. Climb it ladder-style, without your feet.

Planning the layout of your gym

Now that you have thought about your main climbing features, you are ready to start planning the layout of your gym. A large gym will consist of several main features with transition walls (or roofs) between them. Decide what type of main climbing

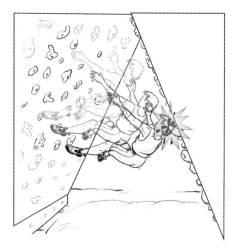

2-13. Place opposing walls too close together and you risk banging your head on a hold when you fall.

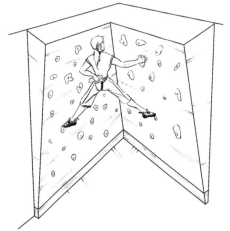

2-14. Stemming corners let you unweight your hands, reducing the effectiveness of your workout. Avoid them.

features you want, and where they should be placed. Remember, the main features will not only influence your climbing, they will also dictate where your storage will be and the general traffic and landing patterns. Also remember the tips in Chapter 1 regarding shade, lighting, and ventilation.

Thinking about your layout. Sit in your empty room, basement, attic, or garage and imagine the climbing walls bending and overhanging around you. Visualize where you will store those bikes, skis, and surfboards. The layout of the climbing surface is only half of the puzzle; the other half is what's behind the walls. Don't squander all that great storage space.

If you are planning a gym in your garage, think about where you will park your car. Maybe the car will be relegated to rotting outside, but this is not necessary. A couple of tips: Don't trap in the driver of a car by placing a very steep wall next to the driver's door. Also, if you are pushed for space, consider making a cave feature to sit over the hood of your car.

Another often ignored aspect of gym design is planning where you will relax and hang out between burns. Your friends will want to be in the center of things while resting, so plan accordingly. Leave them some space where they can sit on the padding without getting hit by a falling climber.

Simulating your layout. Once you have mentally placed the main features, take a thin rope or twine and string it up from floor to ceiling, taping it in place to mimic the angles of your main features. This will show you where these features will intersect and how your gym will actually look.

Use the standard four-by-eight-foot sheet of plywood as the yardstick for planning the width of the various features. It's easiest to frame features with dimensions of four feet, eight feet, 12 feet, 16 feet, and so on. Don't make a wall eight feet six inches wide when you are working with an eight-foot length of plywood. Be careful when you have opposing features (figure 2-13). If you place them too close together, you may collide with the opposite feature when you fall.

Your string outline will also show you the amount of storage space behind your climbing walls and suggest what you might do with it. You don't need to account for all of the space, but you should measure the main items that you plan to store behind the walls. You should also think about how you will access these interior spaces. (See the next chapter for a detailed discussion of storage.)

Transition walls. If everything seems well located at this point, start thinking about the transition walls that connect your main features. If your main features are too close together, you might be able to stem between them and get a no-hands rest — the nemesis of home climbing gyms (figure 2-14). There are numerous ways to mitigate these rests (e.g. triangle inserts and ship's-bow features), but at this stage concentrate on allowing sufficient room (at least six feet) between your main features to create transitions without any vertical or near-vertical walls or corners. Roof sections provide excellent transitions between opposing climbing features, provided that the roof isn't more than 10 feet above the ground.

Ventilation. Now is a good time to mention the use of air conditioning or fans for ventilation. Air conditioning is worth the effort. It not only cools the air, but it also dries it. The easiest air conditioning to install is a window-mounted unit, which can be retrofitted into an existing window. Buy the heaviest-duty air conditioner you can find — you will probably need to run 220 volts to the unit. An easier but less effective option is to install some large fans (these can be set on the ground or bolted to the ceiling).

Lighting. If natural light is lacking, you can install fluorescent lighting on the ceilings. This type of lighting does not give off too much heat. Be careful not to put your lights in locations where they can be hit or kicked while climbing.

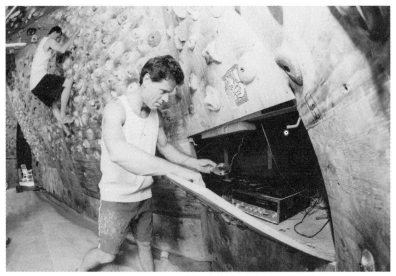

A climbing wall can be as simple as two sheets of plywood screwed to a wall or so elaborate that it includes a sound system – your only limitations are space and money.

Budget and materials

Planning your budget is as important as planning your gym. You won't want to spend $15,000 on a gym in a rental house, from which you may move in six months. Bear in mind that a home gym tends to grow, and the more complicated and intricate its design, the harder it will be to move and fit into a new location. The following tables will help you estimate the cost of your home gym.

Tools

Item	Cost	Number	Purpose
Electric drill	$50	1	Drilling holes, setting drywall screws
Drill bits, 7/16" wood auger	$10	1	Starter holes for inset pockets, T-nut holes (long-bore bit)
Circular saw	$50	1	Cutting panels and studs
Miter saw	$150	1	Makes fast work of cutting studs
Jigsaw	$50	1	For inset pockets
Hammer	$15	1	
Sledge hammer, 2 or 3 lbs	$15	1	Installing T-nuts
Tape measure	$10	1	
Level, four-foot	$10	1	Leveling framing and kicker plate
Chalk line	$12	1	Marking cuts
Safety goggles	$5	1	For all power-tool use
T-bevel	$5	1	Good for measuring angle cuts on studs
Stud finder	$13	1	
Large square (48")	$20	1	Marking T-nut locations and measuring cuts for bending panels
Stanley SureForm	$14	1	Knocking down splinters on rear of T-nut holes
#2 Phillips head screw tips	$2	10	For drywall screws
Grinder tips for drill	$2	4	Finishing pockets
Chemical respirator	$35	1	For working with resin
Sandpaper	$20	1	Selection of 100, 80, 50, 36 grit, for pockets, resin, and plywood
Caulk gun	$4	1	For Liquid Nails
Clamps (6")	$10	4	Holding panels together while drilling T-nut holes, and other chores
Steel bar clamp (12")	$10	4	Temporarily holding panels in place during installation
Allen wrench	$2	1	Tightening holds

The table on the opposite page details the materials you will need and shows a sample budget, based on one four-by-eight-foot sheet of plywood. To estimate the cost of your gym, take this one-sheet budget and multiply it by the total number of sheets you expect to use. I have subtotaled these lists after the cost of the framing, panels, and bolt-on holds; use the remaining list to calculate the extra cost of bells and whistles like inset holds and specialized flooring.

The table above lists the necessary tools and their approximate costs.

Materials list and cost per panel

Item	Description	Source	Cost/unit	Quantity/panel	Cost/panel
Holds/hardware					
T-nuts	3/8" 16x7/16" 4 prong steel, buy in box of 100	Bolt-specialty shop	$0.09	250	$22.50
Bolt-on holds		List in Chapter 11	$6.00	40	$240.00
Allen bolts	3/8" various heads and lengths	Bolt-specialty shop	$0.20	40	$8.00
Framing					
Plywood panels	4'x8'x3/4" CDX	Lumber yard	$17.00	1	$17.00
Wood studs (2x4s)	2"x4"x8' douglas fir	Lumber yard	$2.50	4	$10.00
Wood studs (2x6s)	2"x6"x12' douglas fir	Lumber yard	$5.00	3	$15.00
Fasteners (screws, nails)		Lumber yard	$0.01	50	$0.50
Hardware (hinges, latches)	For storage and access doors	Lumber yard	$1.00	2	$2.00
Angle brackets	For difficult-to-frame sections	Lumber yard	$0.50	5	$2.50
					$317.50
Inset Holds					
Bondo household putty	Thick resin, sold in gallons	Auto-parts or hardware store	$22.00	0.5	$11.00
Aluminum baking tins		Grocery store	$0.40	10	$4.00
Tin adhesive	Liquid Nails	Hardware store	$2.00	0.5	$1.00
Latex gloves		Pharmacy	$0.06	4	$0.24
Silica sand	50lbs, 60 and 120 grit	Specialty store/ sand-blasting materials	$5.00	0.1	$0.50
Mixing containers	Cut top off 1 gal. water bottle		$0.00	1	$0.00
Wooden stir sticks			$0.00	2	$0.00
Electrical					
Electrical	Conduit, wire, junction boxes, etc	Hardware store	$5.00	1	$5.00
Fans	Freestanding or ceiling mounted	Hardware store	$15.00	0.25	$3.75
Lights	Flourescent fixture	Hardware store	$15.00	0.25	$3.75
Flooring					
Rubber matting		Specialty store/ wooden flooring	$2.00	10	$20.00
Carpet padding (used)	3/8" or thicker	Carpet shop, classifieds, etc.	$0.00	3	$0.00
Carpet (used, sq-ft)	Heavier is better, avoid shag carpet	Carpet shop, classifieds, etc.	$1.00	1	$1.00
					$367.74

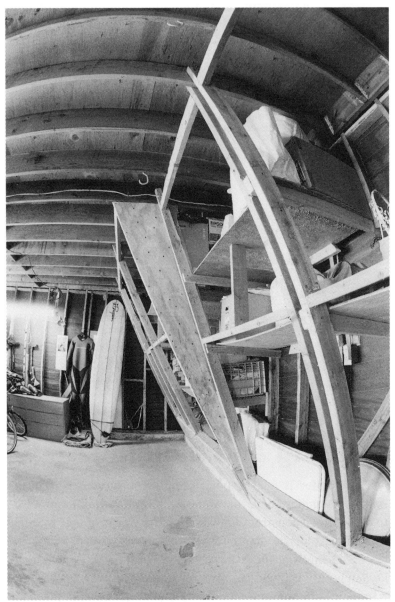

Nothing fancy. If you can swing a hammer and operate a saw and screwdriver, you have all of the skills required to frame a basic climbing wall.

Framing and building

This chapter is for the novice home-gym builder who hasn't swung a hammer since high-school wood-shop class, and needs to brush up on construction basics. A knowledge of how to safely use power tools is mandatory — always read and follow the directions and warnings that come with the tools. Climbing will be much harder if you cut off a few finger tips. If you have construction experience, you might know of better framing techniques than the ones I outline.

Anchors

Wood, screws, nails, and braces. Your understanding of the actual dimensions of wood will be essential throughout the framing process. A two-by-four stud, beam, or stringer may have been two inches wide by four inches deep 25 years ago, but today the actual dimensions are 1.5 inches wide by 3.5 inches deep. Ditto for two-by-sixes or two-by-eights (for all actual lumber dimensions, just subtract a half inch from each stated dimension).

When you are at the lumber yard selecting your framing wood make sure you get the straightest boards. Lay each one end on the ground and hold the other end up to your eye. This quick check will show you which boards are straight and which ones are crooked. Buy the straight ones. Be prepared to cull through an entire pile to find the good boards.

The plywood will attach to the framing via screws. I prefer the drywall screws, or an improved version called Grabbers. These are hard with sharp threads that go into wood without your having to first drill a pilot hole.

Drywall screws come in various lengths; you will want the ones between two and three inches long. You will drive the screws with a reversible power drill fitted with a Philip's bit. These bits wear out quickly so buy a handful.

Avoid framing your wall with nails, which make later wall modifications or dismantling difficult to impossible without severe structural damage. Nails also are a bad choice as they can work loose. Nonetheless, you'll end up nailing in a few tight spots where screws won't reach, or to quickly "tack" studs or other boards into place. Drive them only part way in so that they can be removed when you've finished the attachment with screws. Purchase a couple of pounds of 16d vinyl-coated sinker nails.

While you are at the lumber yard or hardware store, be sure to peruse the bracket and joist-hanger aisle. Here you'll find a variety of metal supports and splicing plates that can help you fabri-

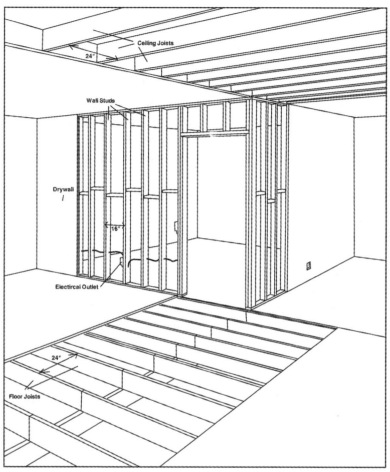

4-15. Modern framing typically places the wall studs 16 inches apart, while ceiling and floor joists are set on 24-inch spans.

cate your wall. I haven't used many of these for my walls, but you may want to, especially if your carpentry isn't up to snuff: joist hangers and angle brackets make easy and strong connections.

Anchoring the wall

After you get your gym design sketched out and the materials purchased, your first order of business is to attach the gym framing to the existing structure. The ideal situation is to have a

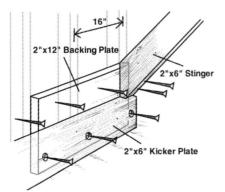

4-16. The kicker and backer plates are the main supports for your wall stringers.

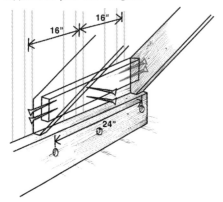

4-17. Eliminating the backer plate creates a less rigid wall, but will still do provided you use cross braces to fortify the stringers.

garage without drywall, as exposed studs provide the fastest and most secure method of attachment. Since modern fire codes mandate covering all walls and ceilings with drywall, you can use a battery-operated stud finder to locate the studs in newer buildings. If you don't have a stud finder, you can usually find the studs by measuring. Studs are generally placed 16 inches on center (figure 4-15), starting at the inside or outside corner of the wall. Electrical outlets are another key because they are generally attached to one of the studs. Once you find one stud, the rest comes easily — knock on wood. Ceiling studs (joists) are generally placed 24 inches on center.

A basic, flat-paneled wall

You will build your wall in a sequence similar to the way you designed it. Start with your main climbing features. For example, if your biggest feature is a 45-degree overhanging wall, frame this first.

Before you get going, though, examine the floor. Is it level? Most garage concrete slabs slope down toward the door to provide drainage. Also check the ceiling to see if it is square and level. Most ceilings (and walls) will be slightly warped or bowed. Don't sweat it; just build your framing to fit as snug as possible.

The first order of business is to install a backing plate, a length

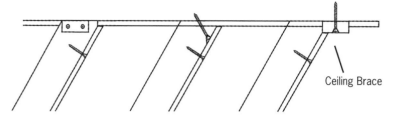

Ceiling Brace

4-18. Three methods for anchoring wall stringers to the ceiling. Left to right: use steel 90-degree plates to attach the stringer to a ceiling joist; angle, or "toenail" the stringer to a joist; and best, screw a ceiling brace to the ceiling joists and let the stringer rest against this.

of two-by-twelve (or cheaper, a 12-inch-high by eight-foot strip of 3/4-inch plywood) to the bottom of the existing wall. The backing plate will provide a solid point for attaching vertical stringers, which form the basis of climbing wall's framing. Screw the backing plate to the wall studs, then screw a kicker plate, a length of two-by-six or two-by-eight that will support the bottom edge of the wall (figure 4-16) to the backing plate. The kicker plate will give your wall a short, vertical bottom section that will keep your heels off of the floor on low problems. If the floor slopes slightly, raise one end of the kicker plate slightly to make it level, and secure this end with extra screws.

Alternately, you can forgo the backing plate and simply have the wall stringers rest on top of the kicker plate (figure 4-17). In this instance you'll attach the stringers to the wall studs when the two line up. Use two-by-four braces to secure the remaining "floating" stringers to the ones that are on the wall studs.

The two-by-four ceiling brace serves the same purpose as the kicker plate but is, of course, anchored to the ceiling joists, the support boards that run through the ceiling (figure 4-18). The distance from the ceiling brace to the kicker plate will determine the wall angle, so measure carefully and use a length of string tacked or taped from the kicker plate to the ceiling plate to check your angle before you permanently anchor the ceiling plate.

If your ceiling joists are exposed, you can omit the ceiling brace and screw the stringers directly into the sides of the joists.

Next, install two-by-six stringers attached at the bottom to the kicker plate and to the ceiling brace or joists at the top. The

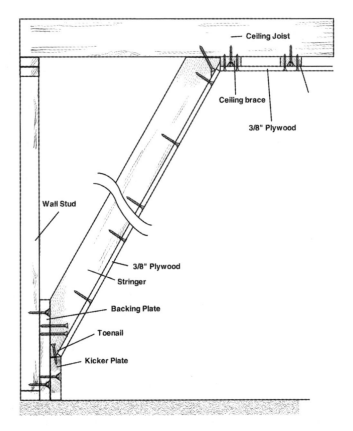

Ceiling Joist

Ceiling brace

3/8" Plywood

Wall Stud

3/8" Plywood

Stringer

Backing Plate

Toenail

Kicker Plate

4-19. Ideally, your wall stringers will be supported by a kicker and backing plate at its base, and a ceiling brace and joist at its top.

stringers form the wall's basic framework, and will determine its angle. Cut one stringer to the correct floor-to-ceiling length, then, with a T-bevel, mark each end with the necessary angle cut. Once you have your first stringer cut, temporarily screw it in place and check to see that it fits correctly. If the stringer is good, remove it and use it as a template to cut the rest of your stringers (you will need one every two feet across the width of your wall).

Screw your first stringer in place at the end of the wall, where the edge of your first sheet of 48-inch-wide plywood will attach. (If you're attaching to a plate, you'll need to "toenail" the screws.)

Screw the second stringer 48 inches away, measuring from the outside edge of the first stringer to the center of the second. When these two stringers are up, hold up a panel to check its fit. The sheet should cover half of the second stringer's thickness, leaving enough exposed stringer to attach the next sheet of plywood. Adjust the stringers in or out or back and forth as necessary. Now add more stringers, each one 48" (center to center for internal stringers) from the last. If you don't have a lot of framing experience, go slow and check each new stringer against the panel before adding the next.

Permanently screw in the stringers, then install more vertical stringers, rib-like, in between the existing stringers at 24-inch intervals. After this, cut horizontal braces and place them between your stringers every 24 inches (from top to bottom). The braces provide more framing to screw the panels into, and stiffen the structure. Figure 4-19 shows the completed framing for a hypothetical section of 45-degree-overhanging wall.

Finally, note that you can install your four-by-eight-foot climbing panels horizontally instead of vertically, if they configure better that way. Generally, however, running the plywood horizontally will not change your framing strategy. Also remember that you need to maintain rear access to all panels for T-nut maintenance — yet another reason to avoid *nailing* the panels in place.

Making the panels

Use 3/4-inch-thick CDX (a cheap exterior-grade) plywood for your panels. Select each sheet of four-by-eight-foot plywood for straightness, lack of splinters, and square edges.

Prepare the panels for installation in mass, and before you screw them to the wall. Stack three to six panels on top of each other, take a power drill with a 7/16-inch bit and bore approximately 250 T-nut holes in a random pattern, or mark off a grid (I do). Either way is fine. If the panels are to be mounted low on the wall, where they'll mostly take footholds, you can get by with half

4-20. A T-Nut setting tool made from a cut-off 3-8-inch threaded rod. Grind one end of the rod with flat sides so it can fit into a power-drill chuck, and use a nut, steel washer, and a rubber washer as your "stop."

the number of T-nut holes. Be careful when the bit breaks through the bottom panel, because it will usually splinter the hole somewhat. For this reason, lay each of the panels with its best side up, so any splintering will be hidden on the back. Next, drill about 15 additional holes along each vertical edge of each panel (avoid splintering the panel and overlapping the stringers by staying one inch away from the edge). Note: you can still screw holds into T-nuts that back onto your framing, as long as the bolt for the hold is sufficiently short.

If you have decided to cut holes for "cut outs" or custom inset pockets (see the next chapter), do so now, before you have attached the T-nuts.

Once you've drilled the T-nut holes, turn over and separately lay each panel face down on a concrete floor or driveway. Using a Stanley Sureform plane, knock down the large splinters, formed by drilling the T-nut holes.

Now, take a light (2 lb.) sledge hammer and tap the T-nuts into each hole. Try and drive the T-nuts straight; you'll have a hard time correcting off-kilter ones once they are installed. If you do get one wrong, pry it out of the rear of the panel with a screwdriver and replace it. Install T-nuts in every panel that you know you won't have to cut very much. But, if you have to cut a panel, leave the T-nuts out — hitting one with a saw is extremely dangerous.

No matter how well you plan, you may later want to place a hold in a location where there is currently no T-nut. A good method for retrofitting T-nuts is as follows. Drill the extra T-nuts holes, then you'll need to fashion a tool for tightening the T-nuts. Cut a shaft of 3/8-inch threaded steel rod (or the end of a bolt), and grind the shank flat in various spots (for the drill chuck to grip on). Next, screw on a nut, washer, then rubber washer. You can now use this tool (figure 4-20) on the end of a drill to tighten the T-Nuts from the outside of the wall as your partner starts them from the inside.

Now that you have your panels drilled and T-nutted, install a few jugs (hand holds) near the center of each panel for handles. The handles will help you maneuver the heavy panels. Get a friend to help you install the panels, because they are awkward and heavy. The hardest panels to install are roof panels. One way to do this job is with three people and a few ladders. Alter-

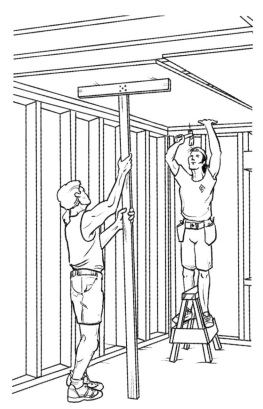

4-21. A T-brace takes much of the strain out of installing ceiling panels.

natively, two people can do it using a T-brace (figure 4-21).

If you're by yourself you can cut the ceiling panels in half; the four-by-four-foot panels are just manageable for one person.

Use drywall screws or "Grabbers" to attach the panels. Drive the screws with an electric drill or electric drywall screw gun. Use 40 or 50 screws per panel, one along every six inches of the perimeter. Make your roof panels even more bombproof by adding a few heavy-duty lag screws. If a panel is warped, start screwing it on at one corner and move progressively to the opposite corner, pressing out the bend as you go.

More Complex Designs

The framing processes for multi-angled walls are similar to those for a flat wall, but more complicated. Before you get started weigh your construction skills and tools you might need to purchase against what it would cost to hire a carpenter to do the work for you. A pro will charge $16 to $20 and hour, and can frame a complex wall in a couple of days. The $300 or so dollars you'll pay him may be less than what you'd spend on tools or tool rental.

Assuming you are game to tackle a complex wall, read on and refer to the diagrams in the previous chapter for details on the framing structure for each wall.

Convex and concave walls. The crux of building convex and concave walls is to get the end angles of the vertical multi-stem stringers cut correctly. It helps to draw the proposed angles on the floor on a piece of long butcher paper. Use this as your pattern to cut the pieces for the stringer. Get one concave or convex stringer right (trial and error, usually), and you can use it as a pattern for the rest. It helps to screw the pieces of each stringer together on the floor, and then attach the assembled stringer to the floor and ceiling braces or joists. As with a flat wall, put the end stringers in place first, and check the fit of the plywood before you fill in the middle stringers. If after completion your wall doesn't feel sturdy enough, go back and retrofit cross or vertical braces at the wall's weak areas.

Stair-step wall. They look complicated but, because the angles are 90 degrees, are actually easier to engineer than concave or convex walls.

Ideally, you'll have the underside of a stairwell to work with, and can simply screw panels to this existing frame. If not, carefully evaluate the difficulty and expense of constructing a stair-step wall against its utility. Unless your gym is three-car-garage-size or larger, your space will likely be better served with simpler designs such as overhanging flat walls. If you do proceed with a stair-step wall, your biggest decision will be its scale: do you want it to run from floor to ceiling, or waist high to ceiling? And what rise and run do you want?

Bending wall. Generally, these walls, which change angles along their width, are best for features that are 16-feet-long or longer. The base of your wall stays the same all the way across (i.e. flush with your residential wall, resting on the kicker plate), while the top gets progressively more overhanging. Once you have determined the starting point for your bending wall (15 degrees overhanging is the maximum starting angle), you will know where your first vertical

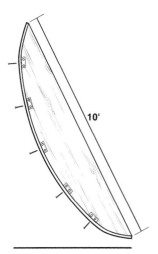

4-22. Fitting plywood to a curved wall requires that you soak the panel to get it pliable. Screw the panel to the wall while it is still wet.

stringer (the least overhanging one) meets the ceiling. Next, determine where you want your last vertical stringer (the most overhanging one) to intersect the ceiling.

Snap a chalk line on the ceiling between the first and last stringer. The chalk line will show you where the other stringers will butt into the ceiling. Finally, fill in your remaining stringers every 24 inches, being careful to measure them correctly. Caution: because each stringer is progressively more overhanging, each will have a different angle cut and length. As with other features, fill in your horizontal braces every two vertical feet.

To determine the shape for each sheet of plywood that will go on your wall, hold a four-by-eight-foot sheet of paper of lightweight cardboard up to the framing, and mark the four sides. Lay the paper on the floor, connect the points, and you have a template that you can lay over the plywood itself.

You will notice that the plywood will need to bend to fit on any sort of curved-wall framing (see Figure 4-22). To make the wood pliable, soak it for several hours. You can spray the panels with a garden hose, or, better, submerge them in a pool. Add the T-nuts *after* the panels are screwed to the framing. Use the threaded-steel-rod method described earlier in the chapter.

Multi-angle wall. This is a lot easier to build than a bending wall, but the result is the same, namely that the wall gets steeper down its length. The big difference with a multi-angle wall is that is has a small arete/corner at every angle change, which gives you an interesting feature. Basically, you build a multi-angle wall by linking a series of single-angle walls, and filling in the transition corners with plywood.

Ship's-bow wall. Start framing with the front of the bow, and work back toward the corners. You can make this feature more complex and interesting by adding more angle changes from top to bottom. The illustration in Chapter 3 shows only one angle change.

Island. Frame an island by first building its long, overhanging side. You can frame this "bouldering wall" on the ground, then tilt it up and use two-by-four bracing to hold in place on the ceiling. After this step, frame your sides and opposite end. An island is like having four free-standing single walls that intersect each other. You can add more interest (and construction complications) by making an island with more than four sides.

In any scenario, be sure to incorporate an access door so you can maintain the panels and store gear inside the island.

Genie. Build your genie on the ground, then attach it to the ceiling joists. A genie is self-supporting; be sure to solidly attach it to the joists. If this box covers a garage-door opener, design it so you can easily unscrew a panel and work on the opener.

Triangle inserts. These overhanging panels go into inside corners where they make stem rests difficult. Correct measuring is the crux to making these features fit the intended space. First, decide on the steepness of your triangle insert; as a rule of thumb, the insert should be at least twice as steep as the steepest wall it intersects. Then, run a string at this angle from the base of the corner to intersect the ceiling at a point midway between the two walls. Draw a diagonal line on the ceiling that passes through this point and intersects both walls out from the corner. Measuring the length of this line and string will give you the dimensions for the triangle insert. Use a circular saw and angle cut the insert so its edges fit flush with the existing walls. Using three-inch drywall screws to attach the insert directly into the corner.

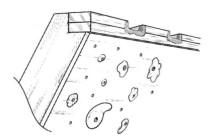

4-23. Roof-line jugs provide positive — and inexpensive — permanent holds where a wall meets a ceiling.

For a more bomb-proof attachment, screw the insert into two-by-four strips that you have preplaced in the corner.

Roof-line jugs. These great features provide a line of buckets where a wall meets a roof. The space around this junction is normally unusable because you can't bolt holds onto an inside corner. Install roof-line jugs during the framing process, and after installing the ceiling panels. To do so, screw a line of two-by-four spacers even with the top of your proposed wall. Next, screw on a two-by-four header, then frame up the vertical stringers to the bottom and inside of that header. Refer to figure 4-23 for details. Finish roof-line jugs by slathering them with polyester resin jelly to form rock-like letterbox slots and pockets.

False ceilings. If your wall is in a garage you'll want to build a false ceiling that lets you open and close the garage door, and use the ceiling space when the door is up. Important considerations for building a false ceiling include sturdy headers that span the room. Use four-by-six headers, and space them no more than four feet apart. When you calculate the height of your false ceiling, don't forget to factor in the thickness of your holds — go too low, and the jugs might scrape the roof of your car.

Free-standing wall. Now that we've reviewed the features some of you might only dream about, we should discuss the only feature your landlord might accept: a free-standing wall. This is the standard-issue bouldering wall with a few modifications. Start by building a flat frame (using two-by-sixes) for the plywood panels.

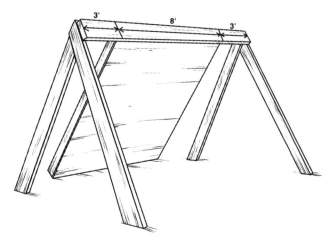

4-24. A free-standing wall is the only structure that won't damage the existing room.

Screw T-nutted panels onto the frame. Next, screw a two-by-eight header across the top of your wall; this needs to extend far enough beyond the edge of the panels so that you won't hit the legs when you fall. Measure the height and calculate the angle cuts for your two-by-eight (or bigger) legs. Raise the wall, using studs to brace it temporarily, and then screw the legs onto the bottom of the header. Presto, you have a freestanding bouldering wall (figure 4-24). If still have trouble with your landlord, tell him it is a piece of furniture.

Storage

Since you need to maintain access to the back of your climbing walls (for fixing T-nuts, etc.), take advantage of the storage space behind your gym. You want to store the most items, while still maintaining organization and accessibility. It's no good having your mountain bike nicely stowed if you can't easily get to it.

Start by thinking about what you need to store. The shapes of surfboards, skis, and kayaks lend themselves to being slid behind a wall. To do this leave openings to the backs of the walls at the perimeters of your gym.

Hinged doors. Hinged doors provide the best rear-wall access, and can also be fitted over existing doors and windows. For good access with the least impact on your climbing, build doors low down on your wall, especially near an inside corner that is not climbed on much. The minimum door size is about 18 inches by 18 inches, just large enough to crawl through. The maximum size is up to you, depending upon what you plan to store behind the wall. I have a three-foot-by-five-foot door in my gym. Heavy-duty hinges and latches keep the door from jiggling when I climb on it. I recommend one hinge for each 18 inches of door height. On the outside, use a barrel bolt every 20 inches, as well as one quick latch. The barrel bolts can be adjusted so the door closes tightly, while the quick latch is for repeated opening and closing without climbing in between.

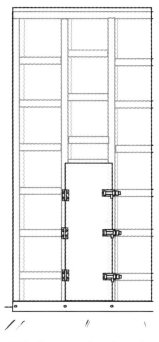

4-25. Plan your door from the outset and you can set it just inside two stringers — simple.

When you cut a door from an overhanging wall, be careful to place it high enough; a badly placed door will swing down and hit the ground, barring entry. Although this may seem obvious, it's a mistake I have made.

Making a hinged door. There are two basic doors: ones that you have planned for during the framing process, and retro-fit doors that are installed after the walls have been built.

A planned door (figure 4-25) is easy to construct. When you are framing your wall, frame a section with your two-by-fours or two-by-sixes that is the size of the door you want to make. If you can place the door at the edge or corner of a plywood panel, you'll do less cutting and half of the framing is already in place. Measure out the corner of your climbing panel where the door is — be sure to have the outline of the door in the center of the framing (i.e. half of the framing overlaps the door, and half overlaps the

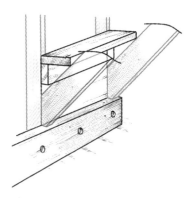

4-26. Build a "catwalk" behind your panels and back-panel access and maintenance will be a cinch.

main panel). This will give the door a natural stopping point and make it stable. Cut out the door section before you install the panel. Install the main panel, then temporarily attach the door panel with a few screws; this will hold the door in place while you attach the hinges, latch, and barrel bolts. Now, take out your temporary screws and you have a working door. If the door panel feels flimsy, you can stiffen it up with some horizontal two-by-four braces, which should be mounted at the same level as each hinge with the four-inch side of the brace flat against the inside of the door.

A retro-fit door also is most easily built at the existing corner of a panel. For this example, however, we'll simulate a more difficult scenario and assume it is placed in the middle of a panel. Trace the outline of the door. Drill the corners of your door with your 7/16-inch bit, then cut the door out, as straight as possible, using a jigsaw. If you are cutting out a section that is on top of existing framing, use a circular saw set to a depth of 3/4 inches so you don't cut into the framing. Next, cut two-by-four framing pieces to border the doorway, overlapping half of the existing wall and half of the doorway. Screw these to the rear of the wall, then temporarily screw the door back on so you can add hinges and latches.

Catwalks and shelves. Since your gym walls tilt at steep angles, walking behind the panels can be treacherous. Catwalks make the space behind the walls user friendly. Attach a few simple triangular supports to the panel backs and frame in a few horizontal planks that you can walk on near the bottom of the interior space (figure 4-26). Your catwalks should be at least six inches wide.

Depending on your storage needs, you may want to build shelves or racks behind your walls. These shelves can actually strengthen your gym by adding more structural framing.

It is easiest to plan and install your catwalks and storage shelves before you screw on your climbing panels.

Lighting. Finally, you need to be able to see within your storage spaces. You can hang drop lights from hooks on the framework, but a better solution is to hire an electrician to hard-wire lights and a switch behind the walls. Be sure to have the switch set near an access panel, where you can operate it without having to crawl behind the wall.

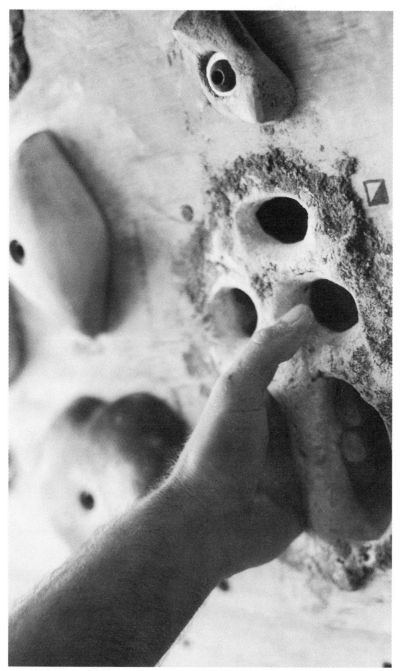

Inset features such as this one are easy and inexpensive to do yourself. Moreover, they add an element of realism to your climbing that you won't get from standard bolt-on holds.

Insets, features, and textures

Some people want to add a textured surface to their gym and make it look "real," while others can't wait any longer to screw holds on the uncoated panels and start climbing. In general, adding texture to the entire surface of your wall is not a good idea. It takes time and money, and makes your wall dark and dingy. Instead, I suggest that you selectively texture the parts of your wall that are likely to see heavy foot use and those where the plywood might splinter (e.g. aretes and corners).

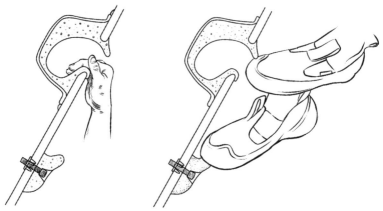

5-27. Inset pockets force you to use real-rock techniques as you must reach into them rather than simply plop a foot or hand onto a protruding knob.

As well as selective texture, inset pockets and features are wall enhancements that all gym owners should consider.

Inset pockets. Making inset pockets (figure 5-27) may seem like a lot of work, but it is worth the effort because they mimic real-rock holds and train those important pocket-pulling muscles. Most importantly, they are usually hard to stand on, and teach you to carefully place your feet, rather than use the sloppy paste-and-push technique encouraged by bolt-on holds.

For this reason, inset pockets make great "starting holds" placed low on the wall. It's nice to have a line of positive hand-holds about three-and-a-half to four feet up from the base of the wall. You can use these holds to pull onto problems from sit-down and crouching starts — the norm in home-gym climbing, since they add more climbing moves to your wall. But imagine a bolt-on jug at the three-foot level on your wall. As soon as you pulled onto the wall you could stand on the jug, thereby defeating the object of making the climbing difficult. Inset pockets are a great way to mitigate this jug/foothold problem.

Making inset pockets. Inset pockets consist of holes in your wall that back onto muffin tins. This space inside the tins is filled with a resin/sand mixture that has been molded into a comfortable finger pocket. The procedure to make them is an art, so it is best to hone your skills on a small, unimportant area of your wall. Assuming that you did not pre-cut the pocket holes, start with an existing panel that is installed on the framing. Using a pencil, draw imaginary one-, two-, three-, and four-finger pockets between the T-nut holes. (If a T-nut is in the way of your proposed pocket location, put it in the middle of the pocket and cut it out with the jigsaw.) Make the holes about 20 percent larger than the actual size of the fingers you plan

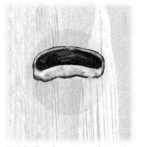

5-28. For finger comfort, give your inset pockets a slight frown shape.

to use in each pocket. You may want to make three- or four-finger pockets with a slight "frown" shape (figure 5-28), which is more grip friendly. Stay away from round pockets — these may look real, but crush your fingers. Of course, there are no rules, and you can make the pockets as challenging as you want.

Once you've drawn the pockets, you will need to drill starter holes for your jig saw. Use the same 7/16-inch bit that you used for your T-nuts. I recommend that you drill at least two holes per pocket, usually at either end.

Always wear safety goggles when using a jigsaw — it's hard to climb blind. Angle your jig saw so that the bottom half of each pocket is cut level with the ground. The bottom of the pocket will then feel slightly incut. Similarly, if you are making an undercling pocket, angle your saw to make the top edge of the pocket feel slightly incut. Once the pockets are cut out, remove sharp edges and splinters with 36- or 50-grit sandpaper. Next, select an aluminum baking tin that is deep and wide enough to accommodate your fingers, without being too large (a big tin requires more work, material, and cost). Mark each tin (on the outside rear) with a number that corresponds to a number you have marked beside each pocket. This is a good idea, since you'll soon be reeling from intoxicating resin fumes.

The resin described in the following section is Bondo Household Putty. There are other resins, but Bondo is the cheapest and most readily available. Wear a chemical respirator when mixing the Bondo. Use one tube of hardener (included) per gallon of resin. Keep the same proportions, even when using small quantities.

Start the resin process by giving each of the aluminum tins a "base coat." This will save you from having to fill the entire interior of the tin through the small hole in the front of the wall. Mix the resin for the base-coat mixture without any silica sand. Using a wooden stick, stir the resin and hardener until it attains a very sticky consistency, like runny cookie dough. Scoop the goo into the tins, and spread it evenly around to coat the bottom and sides. Remove any ridges with your stir stick, because these might abrade your fingers when you are climbing. Avoid getting resin on the rims of the tins. Allow the tins to dry, approximately one hour.

Next, apply Liquid Nails (this is a construction adhesive that comes in caulking tubes) around the rim of each tin, and apply the tins to the rear of the wall, aligning them with their assigned holes. If you plan a down-pulling pocket, place the tin slightly low relative to the hole. Similarly, if you plan an undercling or sidepull pocket, place the tin slightly high or to one side. The viscosity of the Liquid Nails should hold the tins in place until it dries. If the tins start sliding, use a staple gun or duct tape to secure them temporarily. Allow the Liquid Nails approximately 48 hours to dry.

Now you are ready to start creating your pockets. Mix the resin and hardener together (start with about 1/3 quart or less until you get the hang of it), and then start adding silica sand (120 grit for skin friendliness) until the mixture gains the consistency of sand-castle-building sand. Use your hands when the mixture gets too dry to use a stir stick. Wear latex gloves, and have a pan of silica sand nearby to dip your fingers into periodically. This coats your sticky fingers with sand, and temporarily neutralizes the resin mixture so you can continue to work with it. You will need several pairs of gloves — one or two pairs per batch is about right.

Once the resin is mixed, you must work fast because the mix will start to "go off" in about 10 minutes. Grab blobs of the resin mixture, stuff it through the pocket hole, and smear it around the inside of the tin. Carefully fill the inside seam between the tin and the plywood, the inside edge of the plywood where your skin will contact the most, and smear a little bit of the mix on the outside of the plywood next to the pocket. You don't need to cover the outside lip of the pocket greater than 1/2 inch from the opening, unless you are making "hoods", which prevent the pocket from being used as a foothold. Work quickly to use your resin mixture before it hardens. As with the initial mixing, dipping your fingers into the pan of silica sand will neutralize the stickiness of the mixture. When you can no longer shape the resin with your fingers, take rough sandpaper and remove any folds, spikes, or other irregularities. Make the pockets as comfortable as possible. My latest creations at home are as smooth as glass.

Once you have the process wired, expect to spend 20 minutes total on each pocket (that includes drilling, base coat, finish, and clean up). Before you have the system down, you might spend an hour on each pocket with poor results. Start slow, and you will learn how to handle the resin. Speed and perfection will come with practice.

You might have fun making the following types of pockets: mono, two-finger, three-finger, four-finger, smiles, frowns, Star-Trek pockets, Chouca pockets (threads), matching threads, features with hidden holes, sloping holes, underclings, sidepulls, huecos, ball pockets, hourglass pockets, triangles, etc. (see figure 5-29, next page).

Minor features

Minor climbing features are small resin bumps, edges, and smears. These subtle irregularities add a variety to your wall that simple bolt-on holds don't offer. Adding this type of feature is easy. Start by screwing a few drywall screws into you wall, but leave the screw heads sticking out about 2/3 the height of the feature you want to build. These screw heads will form the anchor for your resin. Use a similar mixture to that recommended

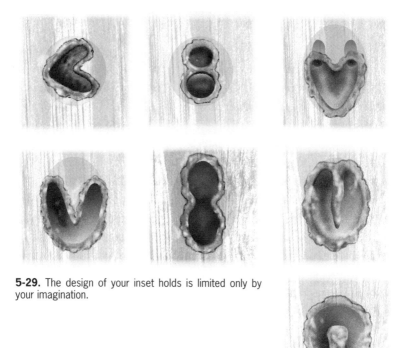

5-29. The design of your inset holds is limited only by your imagination.

for inset pockets, although minor foothold features work better with coarser silica sand (I recommend a mixture of 30 and 60 grit). Bondo Household Putty works OK for the handholds. But for the best handhold-and-foothold results, I recommend Napa Polyester Resin Jelly, because it dries stronger and is less brittle. The Napa resin is twice as expensive as Bondo, harder to find, and more difficult to work with. If you can pay the price and master working with this resin, however, it will give you better and more permanent results.

Larger features

If you want to make larger resin features, make the mixture thicker by adding more sand. Use drywall screws or other hardware to anchor the resin to your wall. Larger features tend to sag while they are drying, so keep an eye on them for the first 10 minutes. Don't be afraid to keep reforming them as they dry. Be bold when making medium features. You can place grapefruit-sized features below roofs and on aretes to add great dimension and variety to your wall. Those of you who are really ambitious can constuct huge huecos and stalactites.

Texture

If you choose to add texture to your climbing walls, do so selectively. Prime candidates for texture are the bottom of your wall, which see a lot of foothold use, and aretes and corners where the plywood tends to splinter. The best material I have found for spot texturing is called Ferrox. This is a two-part epoxy mixture that was manufactured for use on aircraft carrier decks. Part A is a viscous paint with small metal chips in it. Part B is a much smaller volume of epoxy hardener. Unfortunately, Ferrox can be hard to find; try looking in the yellow pages under Marine Deck Coating, Deck Coating, or Construction Supply. If you can't get Ferrox, any two-part textured epoxy mixture should work.

Alternate texture techniques include mixing coarse silica sand with fiberglass resin and hardener. (Fiberglass resin should not be confused with the more viscous Bondo and Napa "resins" described earlier in this chapter.) This mixture can be applied with a paint brush, sponge, or paint roller. You may want to apply several coats. More elaborate commercial-gym-type textures are also available, but remember, most of the texture will be covered when you have finished bolting on your handholds and footholds.

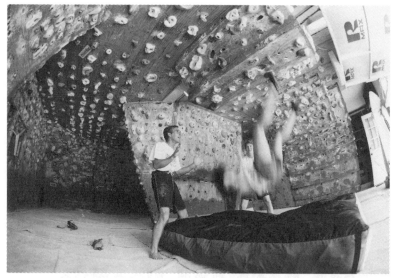

You can't always predict how or where you will fall. Protect yourself against crippling injury by laying a padded floor and placing "crash" mats or mattresses in your anticipated landing zones. Cristina takes a wicked plunge!

Crash pads and flooring

A soft landing area is as important as the holds on your wall, for besides minimizing injury, good padding will encourage you to try harder, maximizing your workouts.

Think about the qualities of the flooring you might choose. Two or three old mattresses will work for padding below a small wall, but for larger gyms, especially those in garages, you may want to walk, vacuum, and even park you car on the flooring. Your padding may also need to be somewhat waterproof — garages can flood during rainstorms, and moisture typically rises through their concrete floors.

Here are some ways to pad the floor of your home gym:

Mattresses. Old bed mattresses protect you reasonably well if you fall on your back, but tend to be too soft to absorb the force of hand- or feet-first landings. You can also injure yourself if you land on the crack between two mattresses or on the edge of one. To prevent this, try stitching your mattresses together with lightweight cord. Mattresses are impossible to drive on, difficult to walk on, and hard to vacuum. Nevertheless, they are cheap (or free), and the most common home-gym crash pads.

To find old mattresses try garage sales, moving sales or giveaways, hotels discarding mattresses, mattress stores getting rid of returns or selling defects.

Carpet padding. You can also pad the floor of your gym with about four layers of used carpet padding (this is the 3/8-inch-thick foam padding used in single layers under carpet). Over that, lay down three layers of used carpet. No tacking down is necessary, just cut the pieces of carpet and padding and lay them on the floor. Tip: cut your carpet from the backside using a utility knife.

For larger gyms, I prefer carpet padding over mattresses, because it is easier to walk on and keep clean. It also provides a nice platform to stretch on. For the real danger areas, though, you will probably still want some well-positioned mattresses or crash pads.

To find used carpet and padding, try the newspaper classifieds. Cheaper still, call some carpet-installation companies and ask if they're getting rid of any carpets and padding from old apartments; they will usually let you haul it (and the cockroaches) away for free. Finally, perhaps you know a carpet installer who can get you some decent second-hand carpet.

Mattress-carpet combo. High-ceiling gyms (10 feet or more) will benefit from having maximum padding all around. I have seen good results with the entire floor covered with sewn-together bed mattresses and then overlaid with several layers of carpet. The carpet layers dull the springiness of the mattresses, which helps prevent injuries.

The deluxe solution. If money is no object you can go for the ultimate floor system: rubber mats covered with carpet padding and carpet, and a selection of gymnastic crash mats. This floor padding is the safest to fall on, great to walk on, and easy to keep clean. It's ideal in garages, because the rubber matting keeps the padding off the sometimes-wet concrete floor. You can also drive a car on the rubber matting and the carpet padding, though you'll prolong the life of the padding by rolling it up between workouts. This may also be safer since any fiber product that comes into contact with your hot car engine could catch on fire.

After you've checked your bank account, go to your local commercial restaurant supply houses or any vendor that sells commercial flooring and ask for interlocking rubber matting with holes. (I purchased my rubber mats from Home Depot on a clearance special.) Purchase enough to cover your entire landing area. Next, overlay the rubber matting with carpet padding and carpet.

Finally, get a few crash pads to place below the areas most likely to see heavy falls. Gymnastic crash pads are best, but new may cost in excess of $1000 each. Sometimes schools will sell secondhand gymnastic pads. Another good option is the Cordless Big Boy crash pad (888-CORDLESS), essentially an over-sized bouldering sketch pad that retails for around $225. The el-cheapo option is to drag in a few old mattresses.

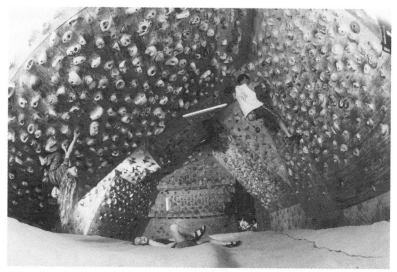

How many holds is enough? The author has 120 per panel, a number that he feels is "just right."

Handholds and footholds

Buying and installing your handholds and footholds is fun. With so many excellent hold manufacturers and designs to choose from, you'll feel like a kid at Christmas. Although you can make your own resin climbing holds, it is extremely difficult and expensive to make good ones — I don't recommend it and haven't included the how-to details here. Wooden holds, however, are practical to make (see the following section).

Choosing handholds

Look for simple, comfortable handholds that you think would be pleasant and interesting to find on a real-rock route. The best texture feels like 80- to 150-grit sandpaper; a rougher texture will chew up your skin, while a smoother texture will feel too slick. Avoid holds that feel sharp, complex, tweaky, or otherwise injurious.

Some companies manufacture inset pockets, but these take up a lot of wall space for a relatively small hold. Instead, I recommend that you make your own inset pockets as previously discussed.

Don't forget to bolt on some good conversation pieces. Many humorous handholds are available from some of the more twisted minds in the industry.

Wooden handholds are cheap and easy to make. They are also smooth and pleasant to climb on, especially at the end of a training session or whenever your skin feels sore. Avoid pine and other fragile woods that can break and send you tumbling. Get some oak handrail, closet-pole end brackets, or small, discarded pieces of hardwood. Cut the wood to size, sand it, drill a bolt hole, and insert a washer. It's as simple as that.

Choosing footholds

Even if you are a beginner, order some small (quarter inch or less), button-like footholds for your gym. Learning to trust these nubbins will teach you the precise footwork that is the trademark of good climbers.

Buying holds. A bewildering number of companies manufacture resin climbing holds. Some manufacturers are better than others, so narrow down your choices by asking your friends for recommendations, and noting the manufacturers of the holds you like at other home gyms and commercial climbing walls. Few retail stores have a good selection of holds, so once you know what you want, call your selected hold manufacturers (see "Where to get your holds," at the end of this chapter). Tell the salesperson what your ability is, how steep your wall is, and what holds you have already. These companies are run by climbers, who can give you good advice. Often, they have pre-packaged handhold sets; these may be earmarked for a certain steepness of climbing (e.g. a set best for 45-degree-overhanging walls). You can also buy groups of holds that are considered better for endurance climbing (jugs) or power climbing (crimps).

Overall, buy a selection of jugs, underclings, pockets, slopers, pinches, crimps, and small footholds. Make sure you have enough variety to train any specific kind of move you find on your real-rock projects. I find it difficult to choose holds from a catalogue, so, again, call up manufacturers and see what they recommend.

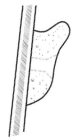

7-30a.

How many holds do you need?

A lot. Estimate the number of holds you think would be adequate and multiply it by five. As a rough measure, consider the bare minimum number of handholds and footholds combined as 15 to 20 per four-by-eight-foot panel. I have 120 handholds per panel in my gym, which feels just right. Now, what mix of holds should you get? A good wall, one that will let you set any sort of route or training routine will have 20 percent of its holds as jugs, 20 percent crimps, 15 percent underclings, 15 percent slopers and pinches, 10 percent pockets, 10 percent positive square-cut holds, and 10 percent small footholds. If you have a lot of roof space, increase the ratio of jugs.

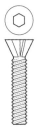

7-30b. No. Avoid holds with tapered allen bolts — the stress imposed by the bolt's flared head can sometimes crack the hold.

Attaching holds to the wall

For the most part, all holds function the same way. They are attached by 3/8-inch allen bolt of varying length, and can be rotated and moved anywhere. I do have a few recommendations: Avoid holds that use a tapered allen bolt (figures 7-30a, 7-30b), which are too hard to tighten. Some people also feel that these bolts tend to split the resin handholds, because they act as a wedge. The Franklin "hardcore" metal inserts have solved this problem. The manufacturer can tell you which of their holds have the taper and which have the standard — and better — allen head or button head (figure 7-31). Most holds come with allen bolts, but double

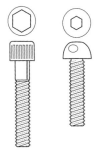

7-31. Yes. Conventional flat-headed allen bolts are what you want.

check. If they don't you can usually buy them separately from the hold company, or pick them up at most hardware stores. Also ask the hold company for an allen wrench that fits the bolts; the type with a "T" handle is the easiest to use.

Fixing up holds

Good quality handholds shouldn't require any work or sanding. Nevertheless, it's worth spending the time to check and prepare your handholds for "skin friendliness" before installation. Fifty-grit and 80-grit sandpaper works well to knock down blemishes and rough spots. Sometimes, you may even want to sand an overly smooth hold to give it a rougher texture. You can use Bondo Household Putty (or other polyester resin) to fill in air bubbles and other defects in holds. Sand the resin smooth after application and hardening.

Now that you know how to patch up sloppy handholds, you may want to buy second-quality holds. Some hold manufacturers sell off holds that do not meet their cosmetic standards. Seconds are often snapped up by employees and their climbing buddies, but it might be worth asking if they are available, since the discounts on them can be substantial.

Where to get your holds

A.S.D. Climbing Equipment
348 King Ave #5
Columbus, OH 43201
(614) 421-1179
(email: AmericaSD@aol.com;
website: members.aol.com/
americasd)

Anatomically Correct / Dyno Holds
522 East Main Street
Meriden, CT 06450
(203) 235-0581

BlueWater
209 Lovvorn Road
Carrollton, GA 30117
(800) 533-7673
(email: bwater@MindSpring.com)

Climbing Dynamics
2706 North 15th Street
Phoenix, AZ 85006
(602) 279-2829

Climb It
3845 S. Main Street
Santa Ana, CA 92707

(714)-751-5038
(714)-540-3845 (fax)
(e-mail: climb-it@primenet.com)

e-Grips
4919 N. Broadway #35
Boulder, CO 80304
(303)-413-0582
(e-mail: egrips@aol.com)

Ent Holds
PO Box 3125
Vancouver, BC
Canada V6B 3X6
(website:www.islandnet.com/entholds)

EntrePrises USA
20512 Nels Anderson Place, Bldg 1
Bend, OR 97701
(800) 580-5463
(email: epsales@empnet.com;
website: www.ep-usa.com)

Franklin Climbing Equipment
Box 7465
Bend, OR 97708
(541) 317-5716
(email:mail@franklinclimbing.com)

GR Holds
678 Indian Road
Windsor, Ontario
Canada N96 2M8
(519) 977-9261
(website:www.netrover.com/
~grholds)

Griphead Wall Rox
5251 Rte 212
Mt. Tremper, NY 12457
(914) 688-7517
(914) 688-7424 (fax)
(website: www.griphead.com)

Groperz
1101 W. 7th St.
St. Paul, MN 55102
(800) 476-7366
(email: SUDITH@aol.com)

Juggernaut
3202 7th street NW
Calgary, Alberta
Canada T2K 1E4
(403) 282-7311
(email: info@juggernet.com; website: www.juggernet.com)

Metolius
63189 Nels Anderson Road
Bend, OR 7701-5739
(541) 382-7585
(email: metolius@empnet.com)

Nicros
519 Payne Ave
St. Paul, MN 55101
(800) 699-1975
fax: (612) 778-8080
(email: sales@nicros.com;
website: www.nicros.com)

Passe Montagne
1760 Montee 2 Rang
Val David, Quebec
Canada, J0T, 2N0
(800) 465-2123

Petrogrips
108 East Cherry Lane
State College, PA 16803
(814) 867-6780
(website:http://users.penn.com/
~petro/index.html)

Pusher
209 West Utopia Avenue
Salt Lake City, UT 84115
(801) 484-1999
(email: mail@pusher.com;
website: www.pusher.com)

Tenze
Bozeman, MT
(800) 971-7818
(website: www.mcn.net/~tenze)

Stone Age Climbing Implements
170 Glenn Way #8
San Carlos, CA 94070
(650) 595-2527
Fax: (650) 596-0407
(email: info@stoneage-gear.com;
website: www.stoneage-gear.com)

Veritech
6666 Deerwood
Cedar Hill, MO 63016-3452
(314) 274-3459
(email:
rinkedinkus@earthlink.net)

VooDoo
2074B Hancock Street
San Diego, CA 92110
(800) 883-6433
(email: voodoo2@flash.net)

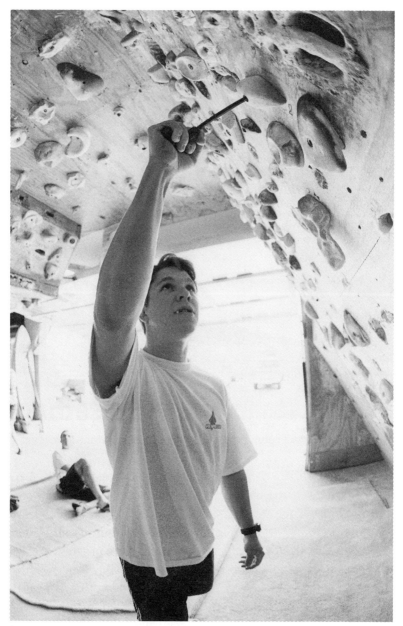

Installing holds is as easy as turning an allen wrench. Even so, you'll likely only move them once or twice a year — give their placement careful thought.

Hold installation, routesetting, and wall maintenance

Now that you've bought your holds you're itching to bolt them on your wall and start climbing. Before you begin, though, it's worth noting that the holds you place will stay put. You'll want to leave your routes and problems more or less unchanged, so your friends can enjoy them and you can measure your future progress and fitness. Aside from minor adjustments, you probably won't want to do a major hold change for at least a year. Given this, it's worth introducing some method to the madness of hold installation.

Before you get going, though, check your T-nuts. Some may be slightly off center in their holes or have their threads clogged with

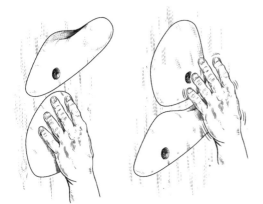

8-32. Set sloper holds underneath your jugs and you'll be able to use both. Reverse their placements and they'll block one another.

bits of wood. Either way the T-nut won't take a bolt and will need repairing either by removing and reinstalling the T-nut or cleaning the threads with a small, sharp-tipped screwdriver or knife.

Hold-installation tips

1. The handholds you place will also be used as a footholds. For this reason underclings are a good choice for your bottom row of handholds. Underclings provide good starting holds for problems and cannot easily be used as footholds. Supplement the underclings with small foot-chips along the very bottom of your wall.

In general, standing on big jugs will not improve your strength or technique. Of course, some big footholds will be inevitable as you climb higher on the wall and you will start using regular handholds as footholds. Plan for this by trying to angle your lower handholds so that they don't present huge footholds later.

2. Don't place all of your holds parallel with the ground. Many holds can be made much more interesting by angling them into underclings, gastons, or sidepulls.

3. Don't group your holds by type. Mix pinches, slopes, crimps, and pockets. This will give you a greater variety of movement options when routesetting.

4. Set some big jugs high on the wall and low down in corners. These locations make good "stations" for starting and finishing problems.

5. Large holds often will affect the way you use other holds. For example, a large jug might cover neighboring T-nut holes, or render a sloper just above it unusable. You can use both the jug

and sloper if you place them the other way around (figure 8-32).

6. Roof sections should be covered in big jugs, right? Not always. Try placing small crimper flakes and pinches on roof sections that are close to an intersecting wall (figure 8-33). You can utilize some otherwise wasted space, and can create many interesting moves this way. Maximize the value of vertical transition walls and arete features by carefully placing tiny slopers and nubbins that would be unusable as handholds anywhere else (figure 8-34).

View your gym as a blank canvas. What you do with your holds greatly affects the flow of climbing and the end result. Imagine your body twisting, turning, knee-dropping, and flowing through the sections. Place your holds with this in mind.

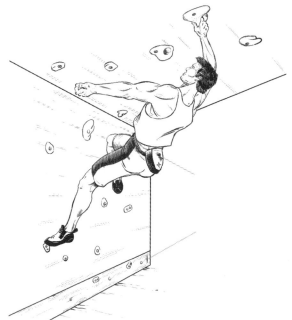

8-33. Place undercling crimper holds on the ceiling, near the junction of the ceiling and wall panels and you can create powerful and interesting reach problems. Keep a crash pad nearby.

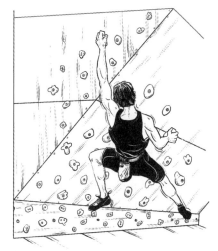

8-34. Maximize small holds by placing them low for your feet and use tiny holds and slopers for transition areas.

Setting problems and routes

Once your holds are installed, you can start setting boulder problems and redpoint routes. Setting boulder problems is straightforward. For example, on your 45-degree wall, find a good low hold (an inset jug or undercling works best), which may be the common starting point for many problems. From this low hold, set five- to seven-move problems that go straight up, traverse, or zigzag. A roof section added above might help you squeeze out a few more moves for the finish. The problems should end on a jug.

Setting good redpoint routes (30 to 160 moves) takes more thought. I look at the big picture before I set a redpoint route, comparing what I am setting to the climbs that already exist, the features it will pass, and the overall flow and feel of the route. How hard do you want to make it? Should you avoid rests? Try setting a route that flows through your gym in a different direction to the existing routes. All of my redpoint routes start and finish at one of three stations. I have strategically placed the stations at good starting and finishing points. I like routes to follow certain themes, like many gaston holds or lots of crimpers. After the first few moves, your route will quickly develop its own personality and may become much harder than you originally intended — that is the nature of the beast. Set routes that challenge your weaknesses. Don't just set routes that feel good because you can do them easily.

To remember the sequence of your route, mark the plywood next to each handhold with a route-specific icon. I do this with a with a colored magic marker or paint. You can start by marking the holds with a pencil, which allows you to easily change sequences before you record them more permanently. If you think you'll frequently change your holds and routes, use colored tape to mark the holds. Alternately you can mark all of the holds with a piece of duct tape, then mark the tape with colored magic markers.

Choose icon schemes that are easily recognizable even when

routes overlap and share holds. A bold red star, for instance, will stand out against a competing scheme of yellow dots or black skulls.

Once a route is set, you can record it in a guidebook using three pieces of information: starting and stopping stations, icon, and number of hand moves.

Route types

"Tracking" problems. Tracking problems use specific (marked) holds for both your hands and feet. These types of problems are excellent for training your weaknesses, because you eliminate big or "trick" footholds that compensate for lack of strength or ability. The disadvantages of tracking routes are that they feel less "free" and you may have difficulty seeing all of the icons and remembering the moves when climbing. For this reason, most of the longer climbs in your gym will be of the non-tracking type, i.e. using specified handholds but allowing any footholds.

No-feet problems. You can do some cool problems with your feet dangling in space. These are a quick power drain and good for developing your stomach muscles and core body strength.

Boulder problems. These are usually five to nine moves long and are marked with tiny letters "A" through "Z". Each problem does something slightly different. For example, "C" features pinches, while "I" features gastons. My circuit took several months to set. Doing "A" through "Z" is a great power workout. I use both tracking and non-tracking problems.

Wood problems. I have a small circuit of problems that just use wood holds. When your "skins hurt," as my Japanese friend Hidetaka Suzuki would say, wood can add hours to your workout.

Circuits. These are short problems that start and finish on the same holds. You can add laps or reverse the sequence. Mine are 12 moves long. If you do two laps, you are doing 24 moves, etc. This type of routesetting works well on small, three-panel walls. Adding laps makes a good, concrete training goal.

Redpoint routes. These are the essence of the garage. My routes average 50 hand moves — the approximate number on an 80-foot sport climb. Many routes are longer (90 to 160 moves), and a few are shorter (30 moves or fewer). These routes are marked with icons. Climbing them feels like a true redpoint. You can milk the rests and choose any sequence you want, as long as you follow the icon handholds. This allows you to be creative and invent improved sequences that the routesetter may not have seen.

Number routes. These routes are like the redpoint routes, but the sequences are determined. The first handhold is marked "1", the second one "2", and so on. Unlike the redpoint routes, number routes need to be followed exactly, with no matching or reversing to shake out. These routes are excellent for endurance training, and, like the circuit routes, can be condensed into a very small space.

Replicating routes. It can be fun and useful to build the crux of a real climb in your garage. This can help you gain special strengths for a specific project, or bring a famous route like *Scarface* (5.13d) at Smith Rock, Oregon, closer to home. The exact replication of routes can be very involved and is a fun exercise to try.

Rules

Rules are no fun, so I believe that it's best to have as few of them as possible. Rather than call it illegal to stem rest in a corner, it is better not to set the route there. The more space you have, the fewer rules you will need. I have only two rules in my gym: First, wood holds are for hands only. This allows you to add more wooden training holds without increasing the number of footholds and making your existing routes easier. Second, hinges and other metal hardware are off limits for your feet. Thoughtful routesetting will help you eliminate rules. Make your wall like real climbing where the rules are simple and few.

Wall Maintenance

It is easy to overlook wall maintenance, but any gym owner will tell you that it is more work than meets the eye. A well-maintained gym is a motivational environment, while a poorly maintained gym is uninspiring and dangerous. A spinning hold, for instance, could leave you with a season-ending injury. The following are regular maintenance tasks that I find useful:

1. Hold tightening: Check and, if necessary, retighten every hold once every six months.

2. T-nut maintenance: T-nuts go bad for various reasons and it is important to have access to the rear of the panels should you need to remove and replace them. When a T-nut needs replacing, say it spins or is stripped, punch it out, insert a new one, but instead of hammering it in place and possibly loosening the other T-nuts, use a hold and bolt to draw the new T-nut into the wood.

Stripped T-nuts that have a hold attached to them can be problematic to remove. Your best bet is to lever a flat prybar under the hold and turn the bolt while it is under tension. If that doesn't work you'll have to hacksaw the bolt.

3. Rearranging the flooring and padding: If you drive cars on your padded gym floor you will need to reposition the padding once a month or more because the cars will twist and move it each time they are driven into the garage. Don't slack off with your padding. If it needs to be moved, repaired, or otherwise fixed, do it as often as necessary. If it needs to be replaced — do it.

4. Vacuuming: A shop vacuum with a nozzle works well to clean grit and dust out of pockets and corners. A stand-up vacuum works well for floors. Vacuum as often as necessary, probably once every two months or after every use if your wall is inside your house.

Like your body, a gym needs regular maintenance. Your new gym will keep you tuned up physically and mentally. Never lose sight of that and you will stay happy.

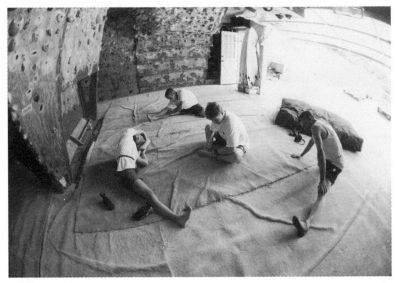
Limbering up prior to another rousing pull session at the author's southern California home gym.

Training

There is a 5.13d called *Riddler*, consisting of a string of difficult boulder problems through overhanging walls, around aretes, and out roofs. There's hardly a rest on this 120-move frenzy, and redpointing it takes as much concentration as any route I've done. The approach to *Riddler* is the easy part. As you might have guessed, it's in my garage, although now you have your own gym, it could be in yours. When you climb on a route like *Riddler*, you don't need to think of it as training — it feels like the real thing. Yet another bonus to working out on "plastic."

Warming up. Avoid sore elbows, torn shoulders, and blown finger tendons by warming up before you really get into it. I suggest you spend at least an hour on the process. Start by climbing on an easy, familiar part of your wall. Make sure you bend and twist your lower body, and don't just pull with your arms and fingers. Do this for 10 minutes or so, then briefly rest. Next, climb a warm-up route that is about three number grades below your maximum ability. Do five or so warm-up routes, slowly progressing to within a grade of your maximum ability and taking a 10- to 15-minute rest between each route. Stretch during your rest time (see "Loosen up," *Climbing* No. 129 for tips and exercises). Depending on your age, body, or available time, you may want to shorten or lengthen this warm-up routine. Don't take too many shortcuts, though, because injuries will cost you more time in the long run.

The heart of your session. With the warm-ups finished, you can get into the groove of redpointing routes or bouldering out problems. It's just like being at the crags, but there are many more things to do between burns. My workouts last between two and eight hours, and I break up the longer ones with non-climbing tasks such as doing the dishes, gardening, and paperwork. I also like to stretch during downtime. At the end of the workout, I like to do other exercises, like sit-ups and leg lifts, to increase my core body strength.

Warming down. It's a good idea to finish off your session by doing several easy routes. This warming down will help to purge lactic acid from your muscles. I also like to do some light weight-lifting exercises, like reverse curls (palm down) or bench presses, that work my outer forearm, chest, and triceps muscles. This helps to prevent injury by balancing the highly developed one-sided "pulling" muscles that you mostly work while climbing (see "Too strong, too weak, or both," *Climbing* No. 174).

Training strategies. Your home gym will allow you to experiment with many different training strategies. When I feel unfit after taking a break from climbing, I find it helpful to start by training endurance (long routes) for several weeks, then gradually shift my emphasis toward power (boulder problems). In general, train power when you feel strongest (after taking a rest day or at the start of a session), and endurance when you don't feel quite at your best.

As a rule, though, there are no rules for training. Do what your body tells you to. Young crimpsters might find that they can flog themselves for hours every day with no down time. Greybeards, however, might only be able to train twice a week. Start slow, err on the side of caution, and add severity or length to your workout when your old one feels too comfortable or boring.

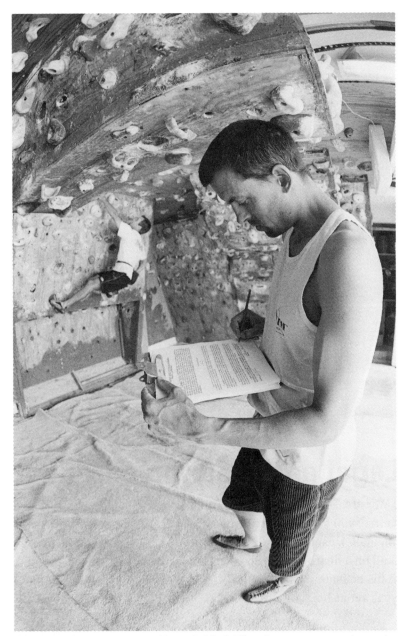

So sue me. Cover your assets with an air-tight liability release — you never know who your real friends are.

Legal and insurance issues

Worst-case scenario: A 16-year-old asks to climb in your gym. Of course, you say yes. He warms up while you go outside to check the mail. Unspotted, he falls from a spinning hold and cracks his skull on a nearby arete. Soon you find yourself next to his parents at his bedside in the hospital. The kid would never sue you, but what about his relatives?

Protecting yourself against lawsuits. We live in a litigious society, so you should think about trying to protect your ass and assets. I suggest you have climbers sign a liability release that might actually hold up in court (see the facing page for a sample). If nothing else, this puts them on constructive notice that climbing in your gym might be dangerous and you are not guaranteeing their safety. I have heard opinions both ways, but the legal theory is that climbing in your home gym is not a necessity for visitors (like food or medical attention), therefore a release is valid because the person signing it is voluntarily entering into the contract for an activity that they chose to do. Minors cannot sign for themselves and need a parent or legal guardian to sign for them. This chapter is merely included to alert you to the problem; contact an attorney for further legal advice. Remember, your first and best defense is proper padding, spotting, and regular hold tightening.

Insuring your gym. You can protect your investment of time and material by insuring your climbing wall. It can be added onto your normal home-owner's policy by simply increasing the building coverage. In general, $1000 marginal insurance will cost approximately $10 per year in premiums. Cheap if, for example, you were faced with a fire that wiped out your garage.

If you are a renter, you probably shouldn't build a wall that is expensive enough to insure — a $5000 wall is a liability if your landlord decides not to renew your lease. Nevertheless, renter's insurance will cover your gym as personal property. Expect to pay roughly $20 per year for each $1000 in coverage. Be sure to have your insurance agent confirm, in writing, what is being insured. As with any insurance, it is a good idea to videotape your insured items and their details. This will help if you need to claim for damage or loss.

RELEASE OF LIABILITY

**THIS DOCUMENT AFFECTS YOUR LEGAL RIGHTS
READ IT CAREFULLY**

I, _____ , AM AWARE THAT ROCK CLIMBING, CLIMBING ON ARTIFICIAL CLIMBING WALLS, USING CLIMBING TRAINING APPARATUS AND PARTICIPATING IN ANY SUCH ACTIVITIES IS HAZARDOUS AND COULD RESULT IN MY INJURY OR DEATH. I AM VOLUNTARILY PARTICIPATING IN THESE ACTIVITIES AT THE HOME GYM OF _____ WITH THE KNOWLEDGE OF THE DANGER INVOLVED AND AM AWARE THAT THE DANGER COULD ARISE FROM MANY DIFFERENT HAZARDS INCLUDING, BUT NOT LIMITED TO THE INADEQUACY OF THE DESIGN, SUITABILITY OR SAFETY OF THE FACILITIES. NEVERTHELESS, I AGREE TO ACCEPT ANY AND ALL RISKS OF INJURY OR DEATH, WHETHER CAUSED BY THE ACTS OF OTHERS OR OTHERWISE.

PLEASE INITIAL

I agree that I will not sue or otherwise make any claim against or their agents or contractors (the "RELEASED PARTIES"), for injury or damage resulting from negligence or other acts, however caused, of or by the RELEASED PARTIES, relating in any manner to, or as a result of, my participation in climbing related activities.

I also agree to release and discharge the RELEASED PARTIES from all actions, claims or demands, for myself, my heirs or personal representatives for injury, death or damage resulting from my participation in climbing and related activities. It is my desire and agreement that this agreement shall fully bind my family, heirs or personal representatives; it shall also be binding as to any other persons, members of my family, including minors, which may accompany me, even if they shall not directly participate in these climbing activities.

In the event that I make any claim, demand or file suit against the RELEASED PARTIES in violation of this Release Of Liability, RELEASED PARTIES shall be entitled to recover any and all actual attorneys fees and costs (including expert witness fees and costs) incurred by RELEASED PARTIES as a result of such claim, demand or suit. This agreement shall be construed in accordance to _____ law, and venue for any action relating to this agreement shall be in _____ , _____ .

I HAVE CAREFULLY READ THIS AGREEMENT AND FULLY UNDERSTAND ITS CONTENTS. I AM AWARE THAT THIS IS A RELEASE OF LIABILITY AND A CONTRACT BETWEEN MYSELF AND RELEASED PARTIES, AND I SIGN IT OF MY OWN FREE WILL.

DATED: _____

SIGNED: _____
(Language for a minor release should be added.)

ABOUT THE AUTHOR

Randy Leavitt, a frequent contributor to *Climbing Magazine,* is one of America's most accomplished and diverse climbers. His ascents range from first ascents of 5.14 sport routes to extreme El Cap nail-ups. Always on the cutting edge, Leavitt has taken to indoor climbing with a fervor that borders on madness. His San Diego home gym has been called "the best crag in Southern California."

OTHER BOOKS FROM *CLIMBING MAGAZINE*

Rock: Tools and Technique $11.95
by Michael Benge and Duane Raleigh
   This easy-to-read, concise book covers all of the ground — belaying, rappelling, protection, leading, equipment.

Ice: Tools and Technique $11.95
by Duane Raleigh
   A popular book for beginners and old salts alike. Tackles the essential topics such as reading ice, staying safe, leading, protection, equipment selection, and all of the tricks for modern pillar and mixed routes.

Quick Clips $7.95
   The best of *Climbing Magazine's* popular column covers tips beyond the essentials for rock, ice, sport, wall, and mixed climbing. 120 tips and 80 illustrations guide you through modifying your ice tools for better stick, to developing one-arm power, to making a bouldering pad, to better knots, and beyond.